MA MAE'S
Healing Hands

Paulette Jones Olasoji

DEDICATION

I my recent years, I, met a woman whom I said, "knows a little about everything". Ma Mae is a woman of value, a priceless jewel in my life. She has shared wisdom and knowledge. I cherish the Wednesday evening talks we've engaged. Ma Mae, thank you for your knowledge of nature's healing and sharing the knowledge with me. To May Bell Arkwright lovingly known as Ma Mae.

Your Spiritual Daughter,

Paulette Jones Olasoji

INTRODUCTION

I was inspired to write this book because of the things I saw my grandmother and great grandmother do that brought back healing. They made teas, poultices and salves from leaves, roots and barks. Great grandma Amy Weston (MA) was a mid-wife who could make things happen with her herbs and teas. Things that we call incurable today were somehow cured with what our grandparents used.

Now I see people fill their cabinets with a pill for this and a capsule for this. I think its time to eat right, exercise, pray and believe God and return to the nature. With this in mind, I set out to capture the knowledge that our ancestors and elderly citizens are taking to the grave because that knowledge is not being written down and passed from generation to generation. So, I present to you:

"MA MAE'S HEALING HANDS"

And by the river upon the bank thereof; on this side and on that side, shall grow all trees for meat, whose leaf shall not fade, neither shall the fruit thereof be consumed: it shall bring forth new fruit according to his months, because their waters they issued out of the sanctuary: and the fruit thereof shall be meat and leaf thereof for medicine." Ezekiel 47:12

My first task in putting together this book was to interview those who tried the naturals and gave overwhelming inspiration of success stories.

My most favorite person to interview was my spiritual mother, MA MAE. Ma Mae lives alone in a small rural neighborhood on the outskirts of Savannah, Ga. I found her to be a wealth of knowledge and experience. I was most impressed with her willingness to share.

As I entered Ma to Mae's humble dwelling place in the country, I found it surrounded with animals and all kinds of flowers and trees. She even had a cotton tree growing in a large flowerpot in her living room. I thought the tree was artificial but Ma Mae said, "no baby", that's real cotton, just feel it. I was like a kid with a new toy. I couldn't believe the plants she managed to grow.

At Christmas she didn't buy a Christmas tree but decorated the cotton tree with ornaments and garlands because the branches were so broad. Every time I entered that woman's house, she told me something new that made me laugh to tears.

I've tried to introduce as many people to her as possible because I've found her to be a rare jewel. Most people who meet her fall automatically in love with and adopt her as their MA MAE. So now I share the secrets of Ma Mae's healing hands and those of others who are willing to share. I've also researched written materials from naturopaths and herbalists to share with people who don't have time to research.

Many of us have gotten used to microwave instant everything; just take a pill and chill attitude. This attitude is causing some of us to live unhappy, and healthy lives.

Others of us are sick because of the cares of this life and our endeavor to get to the top. I believe some of us really need to chill but we don't necessarily need to take a pill to accomplish that.

Many of us just need a daily therapy of Laughter. The scripture says in proverbs 17:22 a merry heart doeth good like medicine but a broken spirit dries the bones.

So don't let trouble and care as cause your bones to be dried but laugh at some of those situations you're crying out about. Doctor bill Gilbert usually sings a song in tears that says God could have given me a lot of things but he put laughter in my soul instead ha! Ha! Ha! Ha! you're probably thinking about your situation and saying it's not funny. Laugh anyway ha! Ha! Ha! Ha!

Those of us who have received the baptism of the Holy Ghost and trust God to do the impossible just need to stand and let God do just that.

Ephesians 1:34 lets us know that the God and the father of our Lord Jesus Christ who have blessed us with all spiritual blessings in heavenly places in Christ according as he hath chosen us in him before the foundation of the world. I believe upon of our spiritual blessing is divine health.

Many people choose prayer and fasting as a method of obtaining the divine health, abstinence of illnesses as well for spiritual upbuilding. This is a fine method, for I believe God does hear and answer prayer. We need to fast with wisdom and guidance as we enter and long-term fasting and breaking the fast. Many have turned their plates down and their face towards heaven and God moved on their behalf.

I have come to find out if we turn another direction God wants that too, we'll find that deliverance we need. Doctor Gilbert, my pastor has taught me that fast and turns us towards God and the reaction he wants us to go, if we fast and pray, Joel 2:12 says "therefore also now sayeth the Lord turning even to me with all your heart, and with fasting, and with weeping, and with mourning."

Some people advocate long fasts for spiritual and health reasons, but wisdom cautions us against long fasting, as they may not be physically beneficial nor a spiritual requirement. Should you be directed to go on a long fast, be sure it's by the unction of the holy spirit as God's bidding. In that instance, don't worry because God has got you covered. If on the other hand this is something you just want to do it would even seem more beneficial to live a fasted life. Short fasts for a few days can be both spiritually and physically more beneficial and cleansing when plenty of water is consumed.

Just abstaining from a diet of rich foods and drinks can be a beneficial fast; and that can safely be done for days and even. weeks. This gives the body a time of purifying itself and resting.

It is not a beneficial fast to abstain from food all day and then in the evening after sundown, eat as much as possible to get ready for the next day's fast. A serious injury to the system can happen when too much food is taken after a fast. This can lead to diarrhea, gas pains and severe cramping. A great deal of the effect of the fast is then lost.

Remember, whatever your reasons for fasting, do it with wisdom and drink a lot of water so the. system can purify itself. If it's a spiritual one, then be led by the Spirit.

There are some foods that are known to destroy the health and should be avoided or very limited in the diet. Some of these foods are spices, mustard, fried, or greasy foods; pastries, predigested foods, coca cola, soft drinks; chewing gum, coffee, tea, cocoa, white flour, salted, fish, tabasco sauce (my favorite), canned meats, condiments, salted meat, Worcestershire sauce, gravies, tobacco, foods too hot or too cold; cane sugar and its products. Our organs have difficulty converting these into pure blood. But wait, that practically empties my cupboard, how about yours?

Condiments make food taste better but are irritating to the delicate lining of the stomach. Mustard and black pepper can irritate the stomach and the skin and ruin the digestive juices. They hinder rather than aide digestion.

Overeating simply tapes the digestive organs, thereby causing impure blood and various diseases. It has been found that over-fed people are much more likely to have cancer than under-fed. Some consequences of overeating are cancer, high blood pressure, Bright's disease, arteriosclerosis and apoplexy.

Only you know your lifestyle. A sedentary life requires less food than an active person. When the bowels are already full, putting a second meal in there just causes the food to be there and sour. Its poisons are absorbed hack into the. blood, and into the system.

It may taste good but knowing when to say enough is enough. Your life may depend on your answer. Those of you who prefer fruit over dessert are doing your system a great service. All fruits have acid that are needed for proper elimination of different toxins, poisonous acids and other impurities in the system.

I can remember my first trip to Nigeria, Africa, no matter what meal was served it ended with orange wedges. Sometimes I would feel so full but the host insisted I eat the wedges. I was told this helped to begin the digestion process. Now I understand why that was such a significant way to end the meal.

A fruit diet can be invaluable, especially during illness or whenever the body has a lot of poisons. A fruit diet will disinfect the stomach and digestive tract. Fresh fruit are more effective. It Is a fantastic cure for constipation and for reducing weight. It is a great source of strength and energy for the body. Eat more fresh fruit and take less laxative pills and oils.

Now it's time to step on some toes. I'll step on my toes first because I love seafood and chicken. But meats of all kind are unnatural foods. Flesh, fish, fowl, and sea foods most likely contain many germs. Meat also house bacteria. It is this bacteria that infects the intestines causing colitis and other diseases. Meat diets most often causes cancer and rheumatism. Excessive uric acid is produced from meat eating and the uric acid causes rheumatism.

Many people who suffer from severe headaches can find relief by cutting back meat in the diet.

I know my co-worker Ruby Peoples would read this and say that meat is an excellent source of needed protein. Ruby is a nutritionist and would agree that the right combination of beans, peas, lentils, and nuts can produce sufficient protein. So, try almonds, hickory nuts, pecans walnut, butternut, peanut, and cocoa nut, and create yourself a healthful protein dinner.

Those who have problems with proper mastication of nuts to prevent large pieces from entering the stomach can use the nuts in emulsified form such as nut butters. Nuts are a very high iron source.

Before we get to preventive methods reportedly tried, I want to reemphasize the importance of prayer, fasting and herbs. The scripture that immediately comes to mind is that of II Kings chapter twenty. That chapter encompasses all that can be taught on the importance of prayer and the ability of God to turn situations around. In those days was Hezekiah sick unto death.

(1) And the prophet Isaiah the son of Amoz came to him and said unto him, Thus saith the Lord, Set thine house in order; for thou shalt die, and not live.(2) Then he turned his face to the wall, and prayed unto the Lord, saying, (3) I beseech thee, O Lord, remember now how I have walked before thee in truth and with a perfect heart, and have done that which is good in thy sight. And Hezekiah wept sore. (4) And it came to pass, afore Isaiah was gone out into the middle court, that the word of the Lord come to him, saying, (5)-Turn again, and tell Hezekiah the captain of my people, thus saith the Lord,

the God of David thy. Father, I have heard thy prayer, I have seen thy tears: behold, I will heal thee: on the third day thou shalt go up unto the house of the Lord. (6) And I will add unto thy days fifteen years; and I will deliver thee and this city out of the hand of the king of Assyria; and I will defend this city for mine own sake, and for my servant David's sake. (7) And Isaiah said, take a lump of figs, and they took and laid it on the boil, and he recovered. (8) And Hezekiah said unto Isaiah, what shall be the sign that the Lord will heal me, and that I shall go up into the house of the Lord the third day? (9) And Isaiah said, this sign shalt thou have of the Lord, that the Lord will do the thing that he hath spoken: shall the shadow go forward ten degrees, or go back ten degrees? (10) And Hezekiah answered, it is a light thing for the shadow to go down ten degrees: nay but let the shadow return backward ten degrees. (11))"And Isaiah the prophet cried unto the Lord: and he brought the shadow ten degrees backward, by which it had gone down in the dial of Ahaz" 2 Kings 20:1-11 KJV Thompson Chain

When Hezekiah heard from the prophet that he was going to die he turned away from everything and began to pray. He brought God back in remembrance of himself and how he had lived. He prayed until he prayed out himself and wept before God. God heard his prayer, saw his tears and was moved by the sight. He was so moved that he promised Hezekiah longevity, fifteen more years of life deliverance and a divine defense. So, we know that prayer works.

Not only should we recognize the power of prayer in this scripture but there was also an herbal remedy for the boil on Hezekiah's flesh.

Isaiah instructed those who served Hezekiah to take a lump of figs and put it on Hezekiah's boil. They did as Isaiah instructed, they "...took and laid it on the boil, and he recovered". You see poultices for the healing of boils is nothing new. If it worked for Hezekiah, shall it not work for us?

No matter what you decide to use be it herbs or prescription drugs, try coupling your choice with prayer and watch God work a miracle in your life. I can say to you as Jesus said, "by faith be it unto you".

Prevention

Oatmeal Water: 2 tsp (heaping) finely flaked oats to a quart of water. Make it stronger or weaker to suit your taste. Let it simmer for half an hour and then beat it with an eggbeater and strain the liquid off. This liquid makes a great drink for anybody but especially the sick. You may add a pinch of salt and a little soybean milk if you desire.

Another Method:

1 heaping tablespoon of oatmeal to a quart of water. Let simmer for two or two and a half hours in a tightly covered pan, and then strain it. Now this is a most refreshing cooling drink when allowed to chill. Oatmeal has natural antiseptic properties that make contagious diseases virtually impossible to catch.

Some herbs have been found to be helpful in certain illnesses but being a nurse, I don't recommend you try to diagnose yourself. I strongly urge you to seek medical attention to diagnose your illness and use herbs in consultation with your physician for best results. Whether you chose herbs or medications remember prayer and faith in God as a Divine Healer will still be your ultimate cure.

With this in mind I urge you to keep your spirit healed and well fed with the word of God and meditation with God on being whole.

Asthma

I think my mother swears by cod liver oil as a cure for asthma. She calls it "fattening the lungs". I can remember having to take cod liver oil as a child. That was our fall tonic to get us prepared for the winter season of colds and flu. I thank God for whoever invented cod liver oil tablets. This has saved many children from the other end of the belt. Two cod liver oil tablets in the morning and two at night is supposed to help prevent colds, flu and asthma attacks.

Tonic herbs work well for asthma. Some herbs can be combined to give even better results. You can mix equal parts of lobelia, wild cherry bark, scull cup, gentian, valerian, calamus, and cubeb berries. Mix completely and use a heaping teaspoonful to a cup of boiling water. Drink one cup three or four times a day one hour before meals, and a cup at bedtime.

Other herbs that can be used for a tea for asthma are hyssop, vervain, skunk-cabbage, colts' foot, mullein, horehound. poplar, black cohosh, yerba Santa, milk-weed jaborandi, bone set, chick weed, lung wort, master wort, pleurisy root, thyme, blue cohosh, calamus, and cubeb berries. Just as above, you can choose two or more of these herbs and mix in equals the mixture one teaspoon to one cup of water one hour before meals and at bedtime. For children give a lesser amount and make the tea even weaker for more frequent ingestion.

An antispasmodic tincture is also valuable along with an herbal cough formula.

Food eaten during asthma attacks can be very important Try simple, non-stimulating and nourishing foods. Have the heaviest meal in the middle of the day and your lighter lunch meal in the evening. A fruit diet for two to three days is also very helpful. After the fruit diet, try light nourishing meals.

Keep the bowels moving regularly at least two to three movements a day. Frequent baths, deep breathing and plenty of outdoor exercise also proves helpful. Make sure your bedroom is well ventilated.

Poor Circulation

Herbs that have proven beneficial to increase circulation are spearmint, catnip, peppermint, vervain, valerian, rue, Colombo, scull cup and gentian root. African red pepper which can be found in capsule form can also help when taken four times a day.

If need be, empty the bowels by using an enema. Do deep breathing exercises morning and evening and regularly during the day, along with plenty of outdoor exercises. Eliminate constipation by using cleansing diets and herbal laxatives.

I dare not leave out exercise. Sedentary living increases pooling of blood to already sluggish veins. If you must sit for long periods, practice proper body alignment and moving as many joints as possible to increase blood flow to all areas. Eat a light lunch and then take a brisk walk. You will surely feel more revived.

Constipation

The first time I met a young woman who told me she had a bowel movement three to five times a month, I was horrified. She was about twenty-eight and she had been that way all her life, so she felt it was normal. I started encouraging water, fruit and vegetables in her diet to ease elimination.

To disinfect and stimulate the colon to bring back good peristalsis, high enemas can be used. Use high enemas made of raspberry leaves, wild cherry bark or leaves, or bay berry bark. Mix one heaping teaspoon to 6 quart of water.

Eat plenty of fresh and stewed fruits as apples, figs. oranges, bananas, blue berries and peaches. Some people are sensitive to certain fruits so choose the ones that suit you best. Train the bowels to move freely, by going to the bathroom after meals and around the same times every day. Bran and oat meals are effective means to make the bowels move. They can be used in cooking, baking or alone. Ifa laxative is needed, mix one tablespoon each of mandrake, buck thorn bark, rhubarb root, fennel seed, calamus root and one teaspoon of aloes.

I can never say enough about water. Drink six-to-eight-ounce glasses of water daily. If you don't like the taste of plain water, keep chilled a squeeze a little lemon juice in it. That gives it a cool, refreshing taste. You can drink a lot of things but there is no real substitute for water. Please get a glass of water right now and let this be the beginning for the rest of your life.

Colitis

A high enema made of one table spoonful of bay berry bark to a quart of water is helpful. Other herbs with great healing properties are yellow dock and burdock root. These can be covered and simmer for a few minutes.

Sleep for fifteen or twenty minutes and then pour off the tea and take as hot as you can stand it. Wild alum root, golden seal and myrrh are also good for use as an enema. Use one teaspoon of golden seal with one teaspoon of myrrh to four quarts of boiling water. Steep and use after the mixture settles.

Just for a few days, a liquid diet may be very beneficial. Chew all solid foods completely avoiding liquids with diet. Avoid roughage and foods containing skins and seeds until condition improves.

Besides those herbs used in high enemas there are also some that are beneficial when taken orally. You can use a fourth teaspoon of golden seal to a pint of boiling water. Let it steep and take one tablespoon of recipe about six to eight times a day. In very severe cases you can take one tablespoon every hour.

Please remember what we said in the outset about irritant like pepper condiments, those things we love so well. They may taste good but they are not necessarily good for you. They are even worse for you if you have colitis.

Cancer

Many of our elders found and successfully used non-poisonous herbs that will heal cancerous sores, both internally and externally.

Most people give in and give up when they hear the diagnosis cancer. For so long cancer has been thought to mean the end to one's life so many people just give in and tire of the struggle.

I usually equate this with the aging process. We try every new thing on the market to fight the aging process but when it comes to fighting cancer, some just lay dormant and die.

The elders found that they had too much to live for so they kept on living. They found that violet leaves or the whole plant had been beneficial in retarding cancer when poor diet habits and other body insulting habits were corrected.

So, before you give up and roll over waiting for the death angel let's try this.

Make a tea of the violet leaves using one half ounce of leaves to a pint of boiling water. Steep tea for half an hour and drink a cup every two hours. A piece of cloth dipped into some of the tea and applied warm over the affected area is helpful. Leave cloth in place until it dries.

A poultice made of fresh violet leaves steeped in boiling water for thirty minutes with added linseed meat is beneficial. As an enema use one ounce of tea to a pint of water and use morning and night. Agrimony and ground ivy are also useful to dry up and heal cancers.

Some excellent herbs for cancer are red clover blossoms, burdock root, yellow dock root, blue violet (the whole plant), golden seal root, gum myrrh, echinacea, aloes, blue flag, gravel root, blood root, dandelion root, African cayenne chickweed, rock rose, agrimony, and Oregon grape.

Mr. Kloss in his treatment of cancer patients used along with herbs nutritious diets. I would like to quote from Mr. Kloss: "The first step to treating cancer is to cleanse the blood stream by thoroughly relieving constipation and making all the organs of elimination active skin, lungs, liver, kidneys, and bowels, and keeping them active. For constipation take herbal laxatives. Use high enemas to cure the colon of any bad condition there. It is necessary to take a fruit diet of orange, grapefruit, lemons, apples, cranberries, unsweetened blue berries, red raspberries, cherries, peaches, pears, ripe strawberries, avocados, pineapples and tomatoes. All fruit should be well ripened on the tree or vine to be fully beneficial.

Tomatoes should be eaten by themselves - not with other foods. Make them a meal. For the first ten days it is advisable to take nothing but unsweetened fruit juices, preferably orange, grapefruit, pineapples, lemon or grape. Do not mix the juice but take different ones at different times. Vegetable juices are very useful also - celery, cucumbers, parsley, lettuce and carrot. Carrot juice is especially valuable in cancer trouble. Drink six glasses of fruit juices a day and six glasses of herbs a day. If you can take more, so much the better. If the herbs are taken in capsules, take number 00 size capsules for a dose (fill capsules full), followed by a glass of hot water, as hot as can be taken readily Take the herbs one hour before taking any fruit juice. Get plenty of exercise and fresh air outdoors in the sunshine. Back to Eden pp 454.

Drink plenty of red clover tea. Drink in place of water. The tea may be made by using a handful of dried blossoms to a quart of cold water. Let it come to a boil and simmer for fifteen minutes. Let it sit covered up until cool enough to drink; then strain, and drink as many glasses a day as you possibly can. Please don't give up until you give God a chance. Remember, there is life and death in the power of the tongue

While you are healing stay away from negative people who drop negative talk and gossip in your spirit, this will impede your progress. Speak positively, think positively and be a positive miracle.

Diarrhea

Diarrhea is usually a product of bacteria, viruses and stress. Watch what you eat, drink and how you live.

Herbs can help with diarrhea as well. Take equal parts of slippery elm, lady's slipper, gentian, wild yam, bay berry bark and scull cup, mixing thoroughly. Use one teaspoon to a cup of boiling water, steep an hour and a half, drink a half cup every half hour until relieved, and then three or. four cups a day. Adding calamus root will prevent griping, fermentation and gas. Other herb combination that can be effectively used are equal parts red raspberry leaves and witch-hazel leaves. Mix together and use a teaspoon to a quart of boiling water, and drink. four or five cups a day as warm as possible. Also give a high enema using either white oak bark, bay berry bark or wild alum root tea. Give the enemas hot as can be tolerated.

Give hot fomentations to the abdomen and spine, ats continuing for half hour, and if a severe case give three or four times a day.

Have a light diet and drink oatmeal water and at least e pint of slippery elm water and barley water.

Eczema

Sometimes dry, itchy patches on the skin can be very annoying Usually it's easy to buy an anti-itch remedy over the counter but this helps only for a short period of time. Some have tried topical steroids that may help.

Our elders found that golden seal, willow, poplar, yellow dock, blue violet, strawberry leaves, or iganum, cleavers and plantain are excellent as teas.

Take equal parts of bur dock root, yellow dock, yarrow, and marsh allow, use a teaspoon of the mixture to a cup of boiling water, steep, strain and drink one half cup four or five times a day Also bathe affected area with tea as well. Do not use soap and water for cleansing, use boric acid solution.

Earache

How many times have your children gone swimming or caught a cold and started with complaint of earache? I know probably to many to remember. This is what our elders did and it worked. Apply heat over the ear and around the neck for relief, prepare a hot foot bath adding a tablespoon of mustard to the bath. Bake a big onion, yes onion, until soft and tie it over the ear.

This will relieve severe pain. Lobelia or slippery elm poultice is very useful for relieving inflammation and pain. Use a medicine dropper to inject in the affected ear. Oil of lobelia or Origanum or a tea made of these herbs. If there is an abscess, use warm peroxide to wash the ear out. Repeat this peroxide treatment to clean out the ear before putting teas in ear.

Fever

Fever is such a common occurrence with the young as well as the old. But our elders found a cure for this as well. They decided that you could use anyone of the following herbs make into a tea and drink frequently until the fever subsides. Use yarrow, red sage, cat nip, pepper mint, wild cherry bark, valerian, black cohosh, tansy, chamomile, elder, bone set, willow bark or leaves, pleurisy root, marigold, nettle and lobelia. Some fevers can be broken up by lemon juice a lone diluted in water without any sweetening

Gallstones

This particular one brings a smile to my face because in one of my research it said drink a bottle olive oil and lay on the right side. The oil would cause the stone to slide through the duct removing the need for surgery. Well, we tried it and the pain went away so I can only imagine the elders were right because he didn't have the surgery until about two years later.

To relieve the gallstones, give cat nip tea enema then apply hot fomentations of lobelia and hops over the liver area. Give a cup of hot tea made of equal parts of the following herbs: buck thorn bark, skull cap, nerve root, gentian and hyssop. Use a teaspoon of mixture to a cup of boiling water. Drink a cup of this tea every hour the first day, then four times a day, one hour before each meal and at bedtime. This helps to liquify the bile.

Wait half an hour after taking the tea and then give four ounces of lemon juice or grapefruit juice beaten thoroughly together. After the lemon juice and olive oil, lay on the right side, with hips elevated. This will enable the oil to run up into the mouth of the gall bladder lubricating it and causing the stories to pass.

Well, James, this sounds like what you tried so give a testimony that it works. Speaking of testimony, James stood up in church and testified about how I gave him this recipe that worked. Everybody in church turned around and looked at me. I'm glad it worked because if it hadn't, I'm sure he would have testified that as well.

Back to the treatment, fomentation of lobelia and hops will soothe the pains, and dilate the gallbladder duct, so the lemon juice and oil can pass. Thoroughly massage under the right rib, rubbing toward the center of the body will ease the passing of the gallstone after the fomentations have been applied and the oil and lemon juice solution given.

It helps to go on a fruit juice diet of oranges and grapefruit. Unsweetened pineapple juice is highly effective. Have a diet high in alkaline foods, potassium broth is a great alkaline food and highly nourishing.

Use the lemon juice and olive oil mixture for three days. Take on an empty stomach. Other valuable herbs are a teaspoon of powdered wood betony, or one of milk weed mixed in half glass of cold water; followed by drinking a glass of hot water. Take an hour before meals and at bedtime.

Again, I must stress, watch your food intake. Some of these problems can be avoided by cutting back on meats and greasy fried foods.

Gout

I can remember when I worked at Washington Hospital Center in Washington D.C., the people that came in with gouty pain and joint stiffness and swelling. Some people will listen when you tell them about their diet, others just want a quick fix microwave pain relief.

So, let's start with the diet. The first step is to remove all harmful products, foods, and drinks from the diet. Then, take a high enema of warm soapy water.

Take equal parts of scull cup, yarran, and valerian, granulated, mix thoroughly together and use a teaspoon to a cup of boiling water. Steep and drink a cup an hour before meals and at bedtime. Use laxative herbs to keep the bowels opens. Herb liniment if applied freely and thoroughly rubbed in, will relieve pain.

Any of these herbs will be beneficial; take singularly or in any combination you desire, using a teaspoon to a cup of boiling water. Steep twenty minutes, and take four cups a day, an hour before each meal and at bedtime. These are the herbs: blue violet, burdock, gentian root, mug wort, rue, birch, sarsaparilla, buck thorn, ginger, penny royal, plantain, wood betony and balm of Gilead.

Gas Pains

Peppermint and spearmint tea are helpful in overcoming gas on the stomach. Also, equal parts of calamus root, valerian, with peppermint or spearmint, granulated mixed together. Use a teaspoon to a cup of boiling water, steep, strain and drink a half cup one hour before each meal and another half cup after meals. These herbs can be used in powdered form as well as capsules if easier. "

To overcome the condition and strengthen the stomach as well as cleanse it, take one fourth teaspoon powdered golden seal in half glass of warm water a half hour before each meal. You may also take one teaspoon golden seal, one forth teaspoon myrrh to a pint of boiling water, steep, and take a swallow a few minutes before eating.

The Spiritual Man

We have gone through a lot of herbs and teas to help the physical man, but what about the spiritual man.

If you ask Ma Mae the key to longevity, she will immediately tell you to live right, love the Lord and stay out of other people's business. Ma Mae must know something because she is eighty-eight years old.

I just want to add to Ma Mae's list that of prayer, praise and fasting. We discussed fasting of the book. But may I expound a little bit more.

Prayer

I believe one needs to have a personal relationship, a oneness with the creator. So many times, people go through life searching for fulfillment. They at times think it's in material gain yet when that is achieved the void is still there.

Personally, I feel oneness in relationship with God can fill the void and close the gap. Take the time to meet with God in prayer and meditation. Feel free to sit down and commune with God. I feel one of the first sincere prayers we can pray in our adult life is the sinner's prayer. It goes something like this: God I realize that I am a sinner. I ask you to forgive me of my sins and come into my life. I believe that Jesus Christ is the Son of God, that the died and rose again for me. I now accept Him as Lord and Savior of my life. I am now saved.

Once you accept Jesus as your personal savior you can move on to a more in-depth conversation with God.

Jesus said whatever you ask the Father in my name, believing you shall receive.

Find an appointed time you can set aside to spend with God. Let it be a time of little or no distraction, quality time with God. As you pray, pray the word. Pray what the word says, I know for a fact that God will honor His word.

Don't spend so much time telling God what you want but give Him some praise and thanksgiving. Remember the Psalmist said in Psalm 100:4. "Enter into his gates with thanksgiving, and into his courts with praise: be thankful unto him and bless his name."

When you came to God thank him and praise him for what he has already done and then ask him for what you want. Be honest with God and be honest with yourself.

Remember too, a time of prayer is not always a time of as king but also a time of fellowship with God. It's a time just to bathe in the presence of God, a time to tell him how wonderful he is and how much you love and adore Him.

Give God a chance to speak to you. He does have something to say, so listen.

The word says in II Chronicles 7:14 "If my people, which are called by my name, shall humble themselves, and pray, and seek my face, and turn from their wicked ways, then will I hear from heaven, and will forgive their sin and will heal their land"

If you're in a position where you know your land needs to be healed then follow the word: humble yourself. Just forget about who you are and think about whose you are. Now pray and seek God's face. After that you still need to turn from your wicked wats. If you find it hard to turn then say you turn me lord, for if you turn me, I shall be turned. Do that and expect your healing PRAISE!

So many times, I go to church and hear people saying when praises go up, blessings come down. What really happens when we praise God is that His presence comes down. The Psalmist says in Psalm 22:3: "But thou art holy, O thou that inhabitest the praise of Israel." The Psalmist goes on to say "....in thy presence is fulness of joy; at thy right hand there are pleasures for ever more." Psalm 16:11

Now let's give Him the praise. You can't praise him effectively with your mouth closed. So, open your mouth and tell Him how great He is and how marvelous are the works of His hands.

Some happens when you pray and praise. You automatically break forth in worship and adoration. At this point you may feel a little broken, a few tears may begin to fall. Don't be ashamed, let the tears fall. You men who have been told not to cry in public, it's okay now. You have come face to face with a fortress mightier than you. All you can do at this point is lift your hands up in a position of surrender. You spirit man has now taken over and the flesh is no longer in control. "The Lord is nigh unto them that are of a broken heart and saveth such as be of a contrite spirit. Psalm 34:18. Know that your God is near. He has come down taken residence on your praise. Now look closely at his right hand. I think there is where you'll see the blessings you have been singing about. At His right hand are pleasure for ever more.

When I stop by Ma Mae's house, she can be heard singing at her appointed time to meet with her creator is twelve noon and six in the evening. She is sure to be found praying, praising and worshipping God.

Fast

Go back and read the beginning of this book on fast because people fast for various reasons. Some people teach that fasting for spiritual reasons is unnecessary because of Jesus victory at the cross.

I won't ask you to go against anything your pastor teaches you unless it's contrary to the word of God. I do agree with your pastor. You don't have to fast; you don't have to pray and you don't have to praise.

But for those of us who want more than just a mediocre spiritual life, prayer, praise and fasting is a must. If after years of preaching of being in church you still feel that something is missing that there is another level in God then in corporate these three principles in your daily life. I am here to tell you there is another level in God, there is a greater anointing in God, there is power in God, and yes, the gifts of the spirit are still in operation in the body of Christ.

Most teachers will encourage a prayer life but not fasting and not praise. That is usually because they have not experienced that level in their walk with God. They can't take you to a place in God where they dare not go. Start your fast. slowly maybe start out by skipping breakfast. Designate this as a time of prayer and fastening. The next time try skipping breakfast and lunch. You can drink something hot to alleviate gas formation. Then tried twenty-four hour fast once a week. I still recommend drinking water and please keep your breath fresh.

Be sure you incorporate prayer with your fast or you're just going hungry. Be attentive to God's voice during your fast that you might hear and obey.

Avoid hypocritical fasts. Don't fast that you can then brag about it or that others may pat you on the back. Please don't fast to bring about things that's totally against God's word or God's nature.

"(4) Behold, ye fast for strife and debate, and to smite with the fist of wickedness: ye shall not fast as ye do this day, to make your voice be heard on high. (5) Is it such a fast that I have chosen? A day for a man to afflict his soul? Is it to bow down his head as a bulrush, and to spread sack cloth and ashes under him? Wilt thou call this a fast, and an acceptable day to the Lord? (6) Is this not the fast that I have chosen? To loose the bends of wickedness, to undo the heavy burdens, to let the oppressed go free and that ye break every yoke? (7) Is it not to deal thy bread to the hungry and that thou bring the poor that are cast out to thy house? When thou seest the waked that thou cover him, and that thou hide not thyself from thine own flesh? Is 58:4-7

Now that you know the kind of fast God will honor, you can expect things to happen.

"(8) Then shall thy light break forth as the morning, and thine health shalt spring forth speedily: and thy righteousness shall go before thee; the glory of the Lord shall be thy reward. (9) Then shalt thou call and the Lord shall answer; thou shalt cry, and he shall say, here I am. If thou take away from the midst of thee the yoke, the putting forth of the finger, and speaking vanity; (10) And if thou draw out thy soul to the hungry, and satisfy the afflicted soul; then shall thy light rise in obscurity, and thy darkness be as the noon day; (11) And the Lord shall guide thee continually, and satisfying thy soul in drought, and make fat thy bones: and thou shalt be like a watered garden, and like a spring of water, whose waters fail not. (12) And they that shall be of thee shall build the old waste places: thou shalt raise up the foundations of many generations; and thou shalt be called, the repairer of the breach, the restorer of the paths to dwell in. (13) If thou turn away thy foot from the Sabbath, from doing thy pleasure on my holy day; and call the sabbath a delight, the holy of the Lord, honorable; and shalt honor him, not doing thine own pleasure, nor speaking thine own words: (14) Then shalt thou delight thyself in the Lord; and I will cause thee to rider upon the high places of the earth; and feed thee with the heritage of Jacob thy father; for the mouth of the Lord hath spoken it." Is 58:8-14

Can you imagine all the blessings you been seeking just because you prayed, praised God, did in honorable fast and obeyed his voice can really be yours. And the blessing won't just be yours but also goes to those who are of you. That means your family, your church family, and even the servants of your household.

I know what you're thinking that was an Old Testament scripture. What about a New Testament scripture just for thoughts.

Hear the word of the Lord concerning fasting. 17 "But thou, when thou fastest anoint thine head, and wash thy face: 18. That thou appear not unto men to fast, but unto thy father which is in secret: and thy father which seeth in secret shall reward thee openly. Matthew 6:17-18 KJV Thompson Chain

Jesus also instructed his disciples in prayer and fasting as a condition for spiritual power. This is most definitely seen in the healing of the demonic son.

(14) And when they were come to the multitude, there came to him a certain man, kneeling down to him, and saying, (15) Lord, have mercy on my son: for he is lunatic, and sore vexed: for oft times he falleth into the fire, and oft into the water, (16) And I brought him to thy disciples, and they could not cure him. (17) And Jesus

answered and said, O faithless and perverse generation, how long shall I be with you? How long shall I suffer you? Bring him hither to me. (18) And Jesus rebuked the devil; and he departed out of him: and the child was cured from that very hour (19) Then came the disciples to Jesus apart, and said why could not we cast him out? (20) And Jesus said unto them, because of your unbelief: for verily I say unto you, if ye have faith as a grain of mustard seed, ye shall say unto this mountain, remove, hence to yonder place; and it shall remove; and nothing shall be impossible unto you (21) How be it this kind goeth out but by prayer and fasting. Matthew 17:14-21

Are you so sure in your spiritual walk you won't come face to face with a kind that comes out only by prayer and fasting!!? Should you come face to face with that kind will you have the faith or the power to call him out? Think about that before you give your answer. Your walk, your personal ministry, your church ministry may depend on the answer you give. If you haven't been praying the way they should, if you have never fasted and don't believe in fasting what would you do when that demon meets you in the middle of your great revival message? That's something to think about you know Somebody is still saying after the death and resurrection of Jesus Christ we need not fast. Let's see what the word says.

(14) Then came to him the disciples of John, saying, why do we and the Pharisees fast oft, but thy disciples fast not? (15) And Jesus said unto them can the children of the bride-chamber mourn as long as the bridegroom is with them? But the day will come when the bridegroom shall be taken from them, and then shall they fast. Matthew 9:14-15 KJV Thompson Chain

Okay, let's see if I can convince you with the leaders of the church at Antioch.

(1) Now there were in the church that was Antioch certain o se prophets and teachers; as Barnabas, and Simeon that was called Niger, and Lucius of Cyrene, and Manaen which had been brought up with Herod the tetrarch, and Saul (2) As they ministered to the Lord, and fasted, the Holy Ghost said, separate me Barnabas and Saul for the work where unto I have called them. (3) And when they had fasted and prayed and laid their hands on them, they sent them away. Acts 13:1-3 KJV **Thompson Chain**

I can't convince you to fast and pray, only the Holy Spirit through the word of God can do that. So, I leave with the word of God:

"Sanctify ye a fast, call a solemn assembly, gather the elders and all the inhabitants of the land into the house

of the Lord your God, and cry unto the Lord: Joel 1:14 KJV

"Therefore, also now, saith the Lord, turn ye even to me with all your heart, and with fasting, and with weeping, and with mourning: Joel 2:12

If you have not been taking care of your temple, Ma Mae's healing hands was written with you in mind. I admonish you to do all you can with all you've got and with all you can have.

If you can't see that far into life's future come on by and let me introduce you to two of the elders in my life Ma Maebell Arkwright age eighty-eight and Aunt Lena Knight aged ninety-nine. These two ladies shows no sign of retreat nor a flag of surrender. They are going through life with all they have while giving God the praise.

(17) Because thou sayest, I am rich, and increased with goods, and have need of nothing, and knowest not that thou art wretched, and miserable, and poor, and blind, and naked: (18) I counsel thee to buy of me gold tried in the fire, that thou mayest be rich; and white raiment, that thou mayest be clothed, and that the shame of thy nakedness do not appear; and anoint thine eyes with eye salve that thou mayest see. Rev 3:17-18 KJV Thompson Chain

www.ingramcontent.com/pod-product-compliance
Lightning Source LLC
Chambersburg PA
CBHW030038230526
45472CB00002B/576